Table of Contents

The year 2020 marked the 60th anniversary for medical laser treatments like red light therapy (RLT) and green light therapy, providing a host of evidence regarding their benefits.

Through emitting red, low-light wavelengths through the skin, red light therapy may naturally jump-start the process of tissue recovery and other forms of rejuvenation. It's believed to work in such ways as increasing blood flow and stimulating collagen production.

Red light therapies have come a long way, but do they really work? Clinical studies show that, yes, red light box therapies have certain healing capabilities and medical applications, thanks to the way they positively affect the human endocrine and immune systems.

This treatment is now cleared by the U.S. Food and Drug Administration for conditions like chronic joint pain and slow-to-heal wounds, and in the near future, we can expect to see more approvals as research continues to unfold.

Red light therapy, also commonly called photobiomodulation or low-level light therapy (LLLT), is a therapeutic treatment that may help improve acne, fine lines, wrinkles, alopecia, and other skin and health conditions.

Historically, red light was first used in the late 19th century for the treatment of smallpox scarring. However, the exact mechanisms of red light therapy were not well-understood until recently. A growing

Red light therapy involves having low-power red light wavelengths emitted directly through the skin, although this process cannot be felt and isn't painful because it doesn't produce any heat.

Red light can be absorbed into the skin to a depth of about eight to 10 millimeters, at which point it has positive effects on cellular energy and multiple nervous system and metabolic processes. This type of light is considered "low level" because it works at an energy density that's low compared to other forms of laser therapies.

If you've never heard of red light therapy before, you might already be familiar with other terms that are used to describe this treatment, such as photobiomodulation (PBM), low-level light therapy

(LLLT), biostimulation (BIOS), photonic stimulation or simply light box therapy.

Although there is still controversy over this treatment and more research is needed, according to some reports, there are virtually no known adverse side effects of red light therapy treatments, but there is a growing list of many anti-aging benefits.

How does it work? A 2012 report published in Annals in Biomedical Engineering stated that red light is used in three primary ways: "to reduce inflammation, edema, and chronic joint disorders; to promote healing of wounds, deeper tissues, and nerves; and to treat neurological disorders and pain."

It's been found to help promote stronger immunity and longevity by increasing cell proliferation and migration, as well as modulating levels of cytokines, growth factors and inflammatory mediators.

How Does Red Light Therapy Work?

Maintaining the health of our cells is important. Cells in the body have crucial daily tasks that keep us functioning throughout our lives. Inside our cells are mitochondria, the energy houses of the body. They are responsible for energy production, among other things. By shining red light therapy onto the skin, energy from the light is absorbed by mitochondria, strengthening the cells and making cells and the overall body-mind functions perform more efficiently and effectively. Maintaining excellent cellular health can bring other positive benefits that will impact short and long-term health and may even prevent the onset of neurodegenerative diseases later in life.

What is red light therapy used for? Studies have found that some of the ways red light wavelengths work to improve overall health include:

- Increasing energy levels by promoting release of ATP (adenosine triphosphate) from cells' mitochondria
- Stimulating DNA/RNA synthesis
- Activating the lymphatic system, an important part of our immune system that helps carry waste out of the body
- Increasing blood flow/circulation, thereby helping bring more oxygen and nutrients to our cells and tissues
- Forming new capillaries (small blood vessels)
- Improving natural production of collagen and fibroblasts, important for skin care and joint and digestive health

- Repairing and restoring damaged soft connective tissue
- Stimulating or decreasing inflammation, which helps control our natural healing capabilities
- Lowering effects of oxidative stress/free radical damage, which is associated with many effects of aging

Here's more about the major red light therapy benefits backed up by scientific studies:

Increased Immunity and Reduced Side Effects of Cancer Treatments

Research done by NASA has shown that red light technology can successfully reduce symptoms experienced by cancer patients, including painful side effects caused from radiation or chemotherapy.

Using far red/near-infrared light-emitting diode devices (called HEALS in some studies) has been shown to release long wavelength energy in the form of photons that stimulate cells to aid in healing.

NASA tested whether this treatment could benefit patients with oral mucositis, a very common and painful side effect of chemotherapy and radiation. The researchers concluded that 96 percent of patients experienced improvement in pain as a result of the HEALS treatment.

They stated, "The HEALS device was well tolerated with no adverse affects to bone marrow and stem cell transplant patients....The HEALS device can provide a cost-effective therapy since the device itself is less expensive than one day at the hospital."

Similar HEALS technology is also now being utilized for the treatment of pediatric brain tumors, slow-healing wounds or infections, diabetic skin ulcers, and serious burns.

Wound Healing and Tissue Repair

Light in the spectral range of 600 to 1,300 nanometers has been found to be useful for promoting wound healing, tissue repair and skin rejuvenation, although it does this through a different mechanism of action compared to many other laser resurfacing treatments.

Most laser therapies used in dermatology offices use intense pulsed light to promote skin rejuvenation by inducing secondary tissue repair. In other words, they cause intentional damage to either the epidermis or the dermis of the skin in order to trigger inflammation, followed by healing.

RLT actually bypasses this initial destructive step and instead directly stimulates regenerative processes in the skin through increased cellular proliferation, migration and adhesion.

It may also help treat skin conditions through regeneration of fibroblasts, keratinocytes and modulation of immune cells (including mast cells, neutrophils and macrophages) all found within skin tissue.

Anti-Aging Effects for Skin and Hair Loss

One use of red light laser therapy that's growing in popularity is treating skin conditions and reversing signs of aging on the skin (i.e, wrinkles and fine lines).

Results from a 2014 study published in Photomedicine and Laser Surgery demonstrated both efficacy and safety for red light therapy in promoting anti-aging skin rejuvenation and intradermal collagen increase when compared against controls. Researchers concluded that red infrared therapy "provides a safe, non-ablative, non-thermal, atraumatic photobiomodulation treatment of skin tissue with high patient satisfaction rates."

Subjects treated with RLT experienced significantly improved skin complexion, improved skin tone, improved texture/feeling, reduced skin roughness, reduced signs of wrinkles and fine lines, and increased collagen density as measured through ultrasonographic tests. Patients with rosacea and redness have also found relief using PBM for skin care, even those who are unable to tolerate higher-heat laser therapies.

Yet another anti-aging effect of red light therapy is potentially reversing hair loss and stimulating follicle hair growth, which works in many of the same ways as red light therapy for wound healing. Results regarding hair growth have been mixed according to studies, but at least a moderate portion of both male and female patients have had positive results for reversing baldness/hair loss when using PBM.

Improved Joint and Musculoskeletal Health

RLT is now being used to treat arthritis symptoms thanks to its capability of stimulating collagen production and rebuilding cartilage.

A 2009 Cochrane review of red light therapy for rheumatoid arthritis concluded that "LLLT could be considered for short-term treatment for relief of pain and morning stiffness for RA patients, particularly since it has few side-effects."

Even in those who don't suffer from arthritis but have other signs of tissue damage or degeneration due to aging, LLLT can still be beneficial. As a 2009 study published in The Lancet showed, "LLLT reduces pain immediately after treatment in acute neck pain and up to 22 weeks after completion of treatment in patients with chronic neck pain."

Other studies have found that even when patients with musculoskeletal disorders don't experience less pain from red light therapy treatments, they have a high chance of experiencing "significantly improved functional outcomes," such as better range of motion.

Cellular rejuvenation and increased blood flow due to red light therapy are two key aspects of improving joint and tissue health. Decreasing oxidative damage, which degenerates joints, and modulating inflammation are other ways that LLLT benefits soft/connective tissue.

Improvement in Sleep Quality

The human body requires exposure to natural light that is only found outdoors in order to regulate various biological systems. When we spend all day indoors and hardly "see the light of day," our cellular energy systems and circadian rhythms suffer, leading to issues like poor sleep, fatigue, mood-related issues and weight gain.

If you can't get outside more, RLT is a simple way to expose your body to more natural light. This can help reset your "circadian clock" and aid in the release of melatonin needed for healthy sleep.

Improved Mood

Another way to explain the benefits of red light is through the lens of Eastern medicine. Ask a Traditional Chinese Medicine practitioner how light helps improve health, immunity and recovery, and he or she will likely compare it to acupuncture's mechanism of action:

Light is a form of energy, and our bodies are just big energy systems.

Light has the power to stimulate specific meridian points and chakra zones in the human body.

Red is said to stimulate the first chakra because it correlates most strongly with our survival instinct (hence why it gives us energy and makes us act quickly, in order to motivate us to pursue things like money, food, sex, power, etc.).

Red light therapy research suggests that this type of light can naturally be energizing and correlated with improved moods by increasing self-confidence, positivity, passion, joyfulness, laughter, social awareness, conversation skills and sensory stimulation.

Unproven Claims

Although studies suggest that RLT can provide the benefits described above, there still isn't sufficient evidence available to determine whether it can help treat other conditions, such as cancer, clinical depression and severely compromised immune function.

It's also not the only type of wavelength that offers benefits. As explained more below, you may have better results with blue wavelengths, and even saunas, if you're dealing with skin or muscular conditions.

Similar Treatments

Red Light Therapy vs. Blue Light Therapy

Blue and red light therapies, two forms of phototherapy (which also includes sun lamps), have some similar benefits and uses, although they work in different ways.

The mechanism of action of both is still not entirely well-understood, but it's believed that PBM devices produce light with wavelengths similar to those of blue light lasers only with broader output peaks. (They're less monochromatic and don't produce heat or friction.)

Blue light is more commonly used at home from light-emitting devices, especially for the treatment of acne. It's been found that blue light reaches the sebaceous (oil) glands in the skin and can help kill porphyrins, which are compounds inside acne bacteria.

Red light is believed to penetrate the skin deeper and may also help acne and other skin disorders by reducing inflammation and improving healing.

Blue light and red light can be emitted from tabletop light therapy devices (which are used at home and usually weaker, requiring about a total of 30 minutes to one hour of treatment time twice per day) or from stronger devices used in doctors' offices that work quicker (sometimes within just several minutes or less).

PBM (Photobiomodulation) vs. Infrared Sauna Treatment

Saunas use heat to produce biological effects, while red light therapy devices do not achieve results by heat alone.

Infrared saunas work by heating objects inside the sauna room, as opposed to heating the air itself like traditional saunas. They do this using charcoal, carbon fiber or other types of emitting surfaces to deliver infrared heat.

Heat is a form of stress that can have certain health benefits, such as improving cardiovascular health, detoxification and physical performance. However, the purpose of PBM is to emit light right into your skin to positively affect cells, rather than using heat. These two therapeutic approaches can be combined since they each have unique effects, so don't be afraid to try both.

Each individual will react to RLT somewhat differently. A general recommendation is to try this form of therapy consistently for about eight to 12 weeks.

You can begin with shorter sessions and consider increasing your time once you monitor your reaction. For best results, aim to complete three to five sessions per week for the first one to four weeks.

Risks and Side Effects

Is red light therapy dangerous? Although low-level laser light therapy seems to be very well-tolerated and unlikely to cause side effects, it still remains controversial whether it can help all patients.

One difficulty that researchers have had gathering results from studies on red light therapy is pinpointing which light ranges are optimal for treating different health conditions and different patients.

Certain published study results have found that RLT can cause negative reactions when an inappropriate choice of light source or an inappropriate dosage is used. There is an optimal dose of light for any particular application, and in the case of red light therapy, often lower doses are found to be more effective than higher doses.

What are the side effects of red light therapy? These can possibly include burning, swelling, dizziness, muscle weakness or nausea.

Keep in mind that seeing results from red light treatments might take patience and that responsiveness is expected to vary. Be sure to work with a qualified PBM practitioner whenever receiving treatments and report any side effects.

Although red light therapy is considered a safe treatment, it is important to consult with your healthcare provider or a board-certified dermatologist before starting treatment.

The frequency and wavelength of red light therapy treatments vary depending on the area being treated.

Your healthcare provider or dermatologist will be able to advise on the treatment frequency and appropriate wavelength of light to help treat a specific condition.

Red light therapy is also available via at-home devices that can be used for a small amount of time daily. However, not all devices have clinical studies to back up their claims. Also, these at-home devices are less powerful than an in-office treatment.

If you are curious about using an at-home red light therapy device, make sure it is approved by the U.S. Food and Drug Administration (FDA), and speak with a medical professional before using it to determine if the device is right for you.

Human studies on red light therapy had small sample sizes, so more research is needed to confirm the safety and effectiveness of the treatment for most people.

Your healthcare provider or therapist can suggest other nonmedical treatments to manage your condition. Alternatives to red light therapy include:

Anti-inflammatory diet. Certain foods may help lower or prevent chronic inflammation, which is thought to trigger many chronic illnesses.

Cognitive behavioral therapy (CBT). CBT is a type of psychotherapy or "talk therapy." It is a well-researched way to treat mental health conditions like anxiety and depression.

Cupping therapy. This ancient practice stimulates blood flow, which may help relieve inflammation and treat some mental health conditions.

Acupuncture. Acupuncture has shown the potential to help reduce chronic pain, improve skin appearance, and help people with their mental health.

Red light therapy has been shown to have numerous benefits for exercise recovery. It is important to note that red light therapy is an excellent complementary recovery option. It is beneficial to use red light therapy along with other recovery methods: rest, nutrition, protein, hydration, active recovery, flexibility recovery and listening to your body.

Here are some of the ways in which red light therapy can help support the body recovering from exercise:

Reduces Muscle Soreness and Inflammation

Muscle soreness and inflammation are common after a workout, especially if you have pushed yourself. Intense exercise can cause inflammation in the body and lactic acid build up, which can lead to sore muscles and decreased athletic performance.

Thanks to red light therapy, reducing muscle soreness and inflammation is easy. The inflammation in the muscles and tissues can be reduced by increasing circulation and promoting the production of anti-inflammatory cytokines. The increased blood flow boosts the affected area with more oxygen and nutrients for a quicker healing process. It will also alleviate the associated pain, swelling and discomfort and allow for faster recovery.

Speeds Up Muscle Recovery

Muscle recovery is important to all athletes and red light therapy is great to stimulate the mitochondria within cells to produce more ATP (ATP is the primary source of energy for cellular processes). By increasing ATP production, red light therapy can enhance the energy available for tissue repair and regeneration, thereby accelerating the recovery process.

Red light therapy also stimulates the production of collagen, a protein essential for tissue repair and regeneration. Collagen provides structural support and promotes the healing of damaged tissues, such as muscles or tendons. By increasing collagen synthesis, red light therapy can aid in the recovery of injured or strained muscles.

Increased Blood Circulation

One of the benefits of red light therapy is helping the body release nitric oxide, a molecule that helps to relax and dilate blood vessels. This vasodilation can enhance blood flow and improve circulation throughout the body. Improved blood circulation delivers oxygen and nutrients more efficiently to tissues and organs, promoting their overall health and function. This increased supply of essential resources can promote healing and speed up the recovery process.

Additionally, red light therapy can stimulate the production of new capillaries, the smallest blood vessels in the body. The growth of new capillaries, called angiogenesis, can further enhance blood flow and contribute to improved circulation and removal of waste products such as carbon dioxide and lactic acid.

Reducing Pain

Whether you are experiencing muscle soreness or injury pain, red light therapy will help. It has analgesic properties, meaning it can help to reduce pain and discomfort associated with exercise-induced muscle soreness or injuries. It can also stimulate the body to release endorphins, the natural pain relief hormone.

By alleviating pain, red light therapy can improve mobility and allow individuals to resume their normal activities sooner, facilitating faster recovery.

Improves Range of Motion

Range of motion is an important factor in exercise. As mentioned above, red light therapy can help reduce soreness, inflammation and pain. Because of this, athletes range of motion increases and they can get back out there quicker.

Incorporating mobility exercises, stretching, and foam rolling into your routine can also enhance recovery by improving flexibility, range of motion, and reducing muscle tension.

Increases Endurance

Red light therapy has been shown to increase endurance by improving energy production in cells (ATP). This increased energy production can help to delay the onset of fatigue during exercise, allowing you to exercise for longer periods of time.

This can help improve muscle endurance and reduce muscle fatigue. One study found that athletes who received red light therapy experienced less muscle fatigue and were able to perform at a higher level than those who did not receive the therapy.

Enhances Muscle Strength

After strength training, athletes aim to rebuild muscle tissues with protein. Red light therapy, along with proper nutrition, can enhance muscle strength by promoting the growth of new muscle cells and tissues. With stronger muscles, risk of injury is reduced and performance is increased.

Injury Recovery

It's important to have a good injury recovery plan. Rest from exercise will be key to helping your body recover and help avoid further damage. Using red light therapy to support the healing process will also be very beneficial. As mentioned above, it can help reduce inflammation and pain, increase blood circulation and repair injured tissues. With these benefits, it's easy to see how red light can help during the injury recovery process.

Red light therapy has also been found to reduce the appearance of scars. Even old scar tissue can be broken down when applying red light daily. This is beneficial for scar tissue that restricts movement. When breaking down this scar tissue, better movement can be achieved.

Improved Sleep

Red light therapy has shown potential benefits for improving sleep quality and regulating the sleep-wake cycle, also known as the circadian rhythm. It can help align the body's internal clock, known as the circadian rhythm, with external cues like natural sunlight. Exposure to red light in the morning or during the day can help reset the circadian rhythm, promoting wakefulness and alertness during the day and supporting better sleep at night.

It can also influence the production of melatonin, a hormone that plays a crucial role in sleep regulation. Exposure to red light in the evening or before bedtime has been shown to support the production of melatonin, which can help shift the body into a relaxed state. The red color has a calming effect on the body and can promote relaxation. By reducing stress and anxiety levels, it can contribute to better sleep quality and faster sleep onset.

Additionally, adopting good sleep hygiene practices, such as maintaining a consistent sleep schedule, creating a relaxing sleep environment, and avoiding stimulating activities before bed, can complement the benefits of red light therapy for improved sleep.

When to Use Red Light Therapy for Exercise Recovery

Red light therapy can be beneficial for exercise recovery in a variety of situations. Here are some instances when using red light therapy for exercise recovery may be appropriate:

Post-Workout Soreness: If you experience muscle soreness or stiffness after exercising, red light therapy may help reduce inflammation and promote muscle recovery.

Injury Rehabilitation: If you have a sports injury, red light therapy may aid in the healing process by increasing circulation and reducing inflammation.

Pre-Workout Preparation: Some athletes use red light therapy before exercising to enhance blood flow and oxygen delivery to their muscles, which can improve performance and reduce the risk of injury.

Travel and Jet Lag: Long periods of travel can take a toll on the body, causing fatigue, muscle soreness, and disrupted sleep. Red light therapy may help reduce these symptoms and promote faster recovery.

Chronic Pain: If you suffer from chronic pain, red light therapy may be an effective non-invasive treatment option that can help alleviate pain and promote healing

Best Exercise Recovery Practices

Exercise recovery consists of various activities and practices that help the body and mind recuperate and restore themselves after physical exertion. Here are some essential components of exercise recovery:

Rest: Adequate rest is crucial for recovery. Allow your body time to recover and repair itself through sleep and periods of relaxation.

Hydration: Proper hydration is essential for replenishing fluids lost during exercise. Drink water or electrolyte-rich fluids to rehydrate and support optimal recovery.

Nutrition: Consume a balanced diet that includes a combination of carbohydrates, proteins, and healthy fats. Nutrient-dense foods provide the necessary fuel and building blocks for muscle repair and growth.

Stretching: Engage in stretching exercises to improve flexibility, release muscle tension, and promote blood circulation. Stretching can also help reduce post-exercise soreness.

Foam rolling: Use a foam roller or other self-myofascial release tools to apply pressure to tight or sore muscles. This can help alleviate muscle knots, increase blood flow, and enhance recovery.

Active recovery: Engage in low-intensity activities such as walking, swimming, or light cycling to promote blood circulation, reduce muscle soreness, and facilitate recovery without excessive strain on the body.

Massage or bodywork: Consider incorporating professional massages or other bodywork techniques like acupuncture or chiropractic adjustments to relieve muscle tension, enhance circulation, and aid in recovery.

Cold or hot therapy: Alternating between cold and hot treatments, such as ice baths or hot showers, can help reduce inflammation and promote muscle recovery. Cold therapy is beneficial immediately after exercise, while heat therapy can be applied later to relax and soothe muscles.

Red light therapy: Red light therapy, also known as low-level laser therapy, uses specific wavelengths of red light to promote cellular regeneration, reduce inflammation, and enhance tissue recovery. It can be used as part of an exercise recovery routine.

Gradual progression: Allow your body time to adapt and avoid overtraining. Gradually increase the intensity, duration, or frequency of your workouts to prevent injury and promote long-term sustainable progress.

Remember, the specific components and duration of exercise recovery can vary depending on factors such as the intensity of your workouts, individual fitness levels, and personal goals. It's important to listen to your body and adjust your recovery routine accordingly.

To incorporate red light therapy into your exercise recovery routine, follow these steps:

Red light therapy device

Choose the right device: Our high-quality red light therapy device emits wavelengths between 630 to 660 nanometers (nm) for optimal results.

Timing and frequency: Use red light therapy after your workout or physical activity. Aim for sessions of 20 to 30 minutes per targeted area. You can apply our red light devices up to 3 times a day for healing or 2 to 3 times per week for maintenance.

Cleanse your skin: Ensure the targeted area is clean and free of any lotions, oils, or clothing that could obstruct the light.

Positioning: Position the red light therapy device on
the targeted area..

Start the session: Turn on the red light therapy
device and expose the targeted area to the red light.
Relax and allow the light to penetrate your skin.
You may choose to close your eyes or listen to
calming music during the session.

Move the device: If you are treating multiple areas,
reposition the device accordingly, ensuring each
area receives equal exposure.

Be consistent: Incorporate red light therapy
consistently into your exercise recovery routine to
experience the potential benefits over time.

While red light therapy is generally considered safe, there are still some precautions and potential risks to keep in mind.

Skin Sensitivity

Some people may have a sensitivity to red light, and their skin may react negatively to the treatment. Before undergoing red light therapy, it's essential to consult with a healthcare professional or a dermatologist to determine if the treatment is suitable for your skin type.

Medical Conditions

People with certain medical conditions should avoid red light therapy. For example, those with lupus, epilepsy, or sensitivity to light may experience adverse reactions to the treatment.

Pregnant women should also avoid red light therapy, as the effects of the treatment on a developing fetus are not yet known.

Interference with Medications

Red light therapy may interfere with certain medications or topical treatments, such as those used to treat acne. Before using red light therapy, it's important to consult with your healthcare provider to ensure that it won't interfere with any medications or treatments you're currently using.

Red light therapy can be performed in-office with larger devices, which most body sculpting companies use. However, smaller devices can be purchased for at-home use for other concerns like joint pain or wrinkles.

The light is directed toward or placed on your body, and a session length can vary from 5 minutes to over an hour. It depends on many factors, including the target area, desired benefits, and device size. Weight loss companies state that benefits can be seen after one use, while others promote multiple sessions for up to a year.

Red light therapy emits red light (hence its name), but is typically not felt during a session as it does not emit heat. While we still aren't exactly sure how red light therapy exerts its benefits, research shows that these wavelengths penetrate into the skin tissue and stimulate the production of the body's natural energy source, adenosine triphosphate (ATP)

Research shows that cold laser therapy can release lipids from fat cells (adipocytes), which explains its popularity as a fat burner. Weight loss is actually one of the more well-known benefits of red light therapy, made popular by body sculpting procedures that use this technology to reduce adipose tissue and tighten skin.

RLT increases blood flow, helping to eliminate waste from the body and ensure a well-functioning metabolism. Cold laser therapy (synonymous with RLT) can reduce oxidative stress, which is known to accelerate the aging process and increase weight-promoting hormones. It can also improve collagen and elastin production, an essential component of healthy skin.

While the optimal red light therapy parameters and protocols are still up for debate for many conditions, 20 minutes of RLT every other day for 2 weeks removed an inch from the participants' waist, hips, and thighs in one 2013 study [7]. A second clinical trial replicated the findings with a 4-inch total loss from the hips, waist, and upper abdomen in overweight participants.

However, it's worth stating that many body contouring companies that promote red light therapy for weight loss make significantly exaggerated claims that are not backed up by scientific evidence. Some studies have even shown that it may not have consistent fat loss results (perhaps caused by a lack of standardized protocols). The literature also shows that it may not reduce the appearance of cellulite, if that's the effect you're looking for.

Overall, while it probably shouldn't be used as a substitute for a healthy lifestyle, it's possible that red light therapy helps to boost your weight loss efforts.

How RLT Can Aid Your Weight Loss Efforts

Red light therapy is more effective for fat reduction when combined with exercise. It can improve athletic performance and speed up post-exercise recovery, which could further benefit your weight loss efforts.

And if pain is preventing you from exercising for weight loss, red light therapy can improve that too. It's beneficial for skeletomuscular pain, with research showing that it benefits conditions like:

- Low back pain

- Tendon pain

- Knee osteoarthritis

- Plantar fasciitis

- Fibromyalgia pain

Mental health concerns can create an obstacle to weight loss tools like diet and exercise, and it turns out that low-level laser therapy may help regulate your mood. However, keep in mind that the evidence is scarce, the studies primarily used near-infrared light therapy, and RLT should not be used in place of other treatments like therapy or your current prescriptions.

If you are wanting to try it out, cold laser therapy is a treatment best used as an add-on for burning fat mass from specific areas of the body. Low-level light therapy may also be beneficial for helping to address any barriers, like pain and depression, that are preventing you from dropping the unwanted pounds.

Weight and Hormones: Where Cold Laser Fits In

Red laser therapy also has hormonal effects that can play a role in boosting weight loss efforts. Both acute and chronic sleep deprivation reduces appetite-satiating hormones (leptin) and increases appetite-stimulating ones like ghrelin. Red light therapy can reverse these effects and help to normalize your appetite, ultimately keeping you full for longer.

When combined with exercise, RLT improves insulin and adiponectin levels two important hormones involved in weight regulation, blood sugar control, inflammation, and appetite. Not only do these benefits help you lose weight, but they have significant benefits for your overall health.

RLT for Thyroid Health

If you are struggling with a low metabolism due to hypothyroidism, cold laser therapy may increase thyroid hormone output. One study found that 30% of the participants were able to stop their thyroid medication within 3 months after starting RLT with selenium, vitamin D, and/or iron.

Though the added supplements make it hard to tease out which therapy pulled the most weight, another RLT-only trial showed that half the participants were able to maintain normal thyroid status 9 months after discontinuing their medication.

Those with Hashimoto's thyroiditis may also see the added benefit of reduced thyroid antibodies, but the only long-term study to date shows that they reappeared after 6 years.

While this evidence is promising, it's strongly recommended that you don't stop your thyroid medication suddenly, and follow a tapering schedule while working with a thyroid-knowledgeable practitioner. It's also unclear how long these benefits last, as in the case of TPO antibodies, and not all research supports the use of red light therapy treatments for thyroid health.

There are plenty of other options that are well-proven to support a healthy thyroid, including probiotics, selenium, and vitamin D. We offer a self-paced, online thyroid course if you are ready to tackle your thyroid health today no RLT required.

In the short-term, red light therapy is considered to be safe. Research suggests that it's even safe for use on the head for brain disorders and on the neck for thyroid dysfunction. Keep in mind that more long-term studies are needed to truly show its safety profile.

Most of the known side effects are topical and may include:

- Skin irritation
- Redness
- Stinging
- Skin peeling
- Hyperpigmentation (skin darkening)

Red light therapy appears to play a role in treating unwanted weight gain, but its benefits are not yet well-understood. While it's not a "risk" per se, it's unclear whether it offers sustainable benefits for most conditions, meaning the effects may wear off after use or the body may build a "tolerance" to it.

The most important concern when looking for a RLT device is to purchase one that has been FDA approved. Many companies are now selling cold lasers for half the cost, but may not hold up to their promises. It's essential that the device emits the correct wavelength and frequencies. As both at-home and in-office devices are costly, you will want to make sure you're purchasing an authentic, approved cold laser.

However, once you have a device, the ideal treatment parameters (intensity, wavelength, etc.)

for most conditions can be unclear. Daily treatments can be time-consuming (often the same length as a high-intensity interval training session).

Overall, the biggest concerns of red light therapy for weight loss surround the lack of research on its use and effects. This can make it an expensive and time-consuming treatment that may not provide everything you're looking for.

Is Red Light Therapy At Home Effective?

Infrared Light Therapy at home is just as effective as going to a salon or spa which has a Red Light Therapy Panel.

The beauty of LED Light Therapy is that it is a non-invasive skin procedure. This means the treatment is painless and super easy to do at home.

How to Use Red Light Therapy

You don't need to go to a doctor's office and spend hundreds of dollars a pop for the amazing benefits of red light therapy. Easy-to-use handheld red light devices allow you to experience it in the comfort of your home. Just direct the device over the treatment area and let the penetrating red and NIR light waves get to work.

It's a simple treatment, but there are three key aspects you need to consider to get the most out of your red light therapy. They are the power density, the dose and the length of treatment.

The power density or intensity of the red light is measured in milliwatts per cm2 (mW/cm2) and is determined by the distance of the light from the skin during treatment. Basically, it's the number of light photons hitting the targeted area. An ideal power density is 20mW/cm2. But the closer the light is to your skin, the greater the power.

The dose of red light reaching your cells is determined by the power density and the time spent using the light -- it's measured in Joules per cm2. Research indicates that the optimal dose for the skin is 4-6 Joules/cm2. To treat deeper tissues, a stronger dose of 50-100 Joules/cm2 is needed.

If you know the power density of the light then you can work out the dose you're getting each minute. For example, if you're using a light therapy device (like the one we offer) with an intensity of 20mW/cm2, the equation would be 20 x 60 seconds/1000 = 1.2 Joules/cm2 per minute.

Therefore, when using our BlockBlueLight handheld red light device, you'll hold it 50cm away from each area for 4-6 minutes for optimal dose and intensity. For deeper issues, hold it 5-20cm away from the area for 10-20 minutes for a greater intensity and healing dose.

Don't forget to remove any clothing covering the treatment area before using a red light therapy device. The light may feel pleasantly warm, but it won't get hot and will never burn you.

Alternatively if your wanting to treat a larger area with more power, our Red Light Therapy Power Panel Range is ideal for this. Expose the area you want to treat from 3-6 inches away - treat each area for 5-15 minutes (no more than 20 minutes) 4-10 times per week. Some suggestions on how to use the light are below:

Choosing the Right Light Therapy Device

It's great news that handheld red and NIR light therapy device are becoming more easily available. But how do you know the device you buy has therapeutic benefits? That's a good question!

For maximum benefit, look out for the following:

- Efficient and durable LED lights
- Clinically proven red light waves between 630-680nm
- Clinically proven near-infrared light waves between 800-880nm
- A low electromagnetic frequency (EMF) output

Devices that fall outside the recommended wavelengths, such as 600 or 700nm, will not affect your cells.

It likely won't hurt. Red light therapy is noninvasive and is painless for most people. A handheld device may be pressed against the skin at the site of the injury or pain. If you are lying in a full body bed or pod that uses both red and near-infrared light, you may feel warmth from the near-infrared bulbs. You should not expect to experience side effects from treatment.

Watch your eyes. Ask the practitioner if it's necessary to wear eye protection during treatment.

You may need more than one treatment. Talk to your practitioner ahead of time to understand how many sessions you will need (and how often), so you can fully understand the scope of treatment.

This will differ widely depending on the health concern you're addressing. "In certain scenarios, even a single treatment has been shown to be effective, while the most intense PBM treatment is three times per week for four weeks, minimum, to see a prominent effect.

With all this said, keep in mind that the world of phototherapy is evolving, and more research is needed to determine the best uses for the various wavelengths, doses, and devices for specific health conditions. It's best to consult a dermatologist, pain specialist, or your doctor if you have questions or before you commit to any high-cost treatment. Medical guidance will help you weigh the benefits and risks of red light therapy for your specific health goals.

Red light therapy is an effective therapeutic treatment that has many potential benefits. Recent clinical data suggests red light therapy may help treat muscle pain, inflammation, and acne among other benefits.

While new research is promising and shows red light therapy is a safe and effective treatment, many studies have conflicts of interest or other limitations. More research will be needed to determine long-term impacts of red light therapy on health.